EXOCRINE PANCREATIC INSUFFICIENCY (EPI) DIET COOKBOOK

Delicious-Rich Recipes, Meal Plans And Guidelines To Boost Digestive Health, Enhance Nutrient Absorption, And Improve Quality Of Life

DR. AMARI VALERIE

TABLE OF CONTENTS

CHAPTER ONE 19

Comprehending Exocrine Pancreatic Insufficiency (EPI) 19

Definition And Causes Of EPI 19

Symptoms And Diagnosis 20

The Function Of The Pancreas In Digestion 20

The Significance Of Diet In The Management Of EPI 21

Treatment Options Overview 22

Diet In The Management Of EPI 22

CHAPTER TWO 27

EPI-Friendly Nutrient-Rich Foods 27

Essential Nutrients For Digestive Health 28

Foods That Should Be Incorporated Into An EPI Diet 29

Foods To Avoid 29

The Function Of Fiber In The Management Of EPI 30

The Significance Of Hydration 31

CHAPTER THREE 33
Formulating A Meal Plan For EPI....................33
Methods For Formulating A Well-Balanced Meal Plan 34
Meal Plans Examples 35
Strategies For Meal Preparation 35
Significance Of Portion Control 36
Frequently Asked Questions And Common Concerns 37
CHAPTER FOUR..43
Foods To Avoid And The Reasons For Their Avoidance 43
Foods That Exacerbate Symptoms Of EPI 43
Comprehending Trigger Ingredients............44
Substitutes For Prevalently Problematic Cuisines 45
Comprehending And Interpreting Food Labels 46
Meal Planning And Preparation 47
Methods For Formulating An Efficient Diet Schedule..47

Sample Menu Arrangements For Varying Caloric Requirements 48

Recommendations For Recipe Preparation And Batch Cooking 49

The Significance Of Feeding Timing And Frequency 50

CHAPTER FIVE 51

Recipes That Are Both Nutritious And Delicious 51

Breakfast Recipes: Simple And Rapid Alternatives 52

Lunch Recipes: Nutritious And Satisfying Meals 52

Dinner Recipes: Delicious And Well-Received Meals 53

Healthy And Satisfying Snack Recipes 54

Dessert Recipes: Indulgent And EPI-Friendly Desserts 55

CHAPTER SIX 57

Eating Out And Handling Social Situations 57

How To Manage Social Gatherings And Parties 58

Finding EPI-Friendly Restaurant Options 60

CHAPTER SEVEN 63

Seven-Day Meal Plan, Ingredients, And Detailed Preparatory Guidelines For Exocrine Pancreatic Insufficiency 63

CHAPTER EIGHT 93

7 Desserts Procedural Recipes For Exocrine Pancreatic Insufficiency (EPI) And Guidelines . 93

General Recommendations For Desserts That Are EPI-Friendly 102

CHAPTER NINE 105

7 Smoothie Procedural Recipes For Exocrine Pancreatic Insufficiency (EPI) 105

EPI-Friendly Smoothies: A Guide 106

CHAPTER TEN 115

Maintaining A Healthy Lifestyle With EPI 115

The Significance Of Consistent Medical Examinations 115

Maintaining A Healthy Weight And Engaging In Physical Activity 116

Management Of Stress And Its Effect On Digestive Health 117

Establishing A Support System 118

Monitoring And Modifying Your Diet Over Time 119

Conclusion 120

THE END 123

BONUS:

7 days meal plan recipes, ingredients, and detailed preparatory guidelines for Exocrine Pancreatic Insufficiency (EPI)

7 Desserts procedural recipes for Exocrine Pancreatic Insufficiency (EPI) and guidelines

7 Smoothies procedural recipes for Exocrine Pancreatic Insufficiency (EPI) and guidelines

Copyright © 2024 By Dr. Amari Valerie

All rights reserved

No part of this book may be reproduced, distributed, or transmitted in any form or by any means, including photocopying, recording, or other electronic or mechanical methods, without the prior written permission of the publisher, except in the case of brief quotations embodied in critical reviews and certain other noncommercial uses permitted by copyright law.

DISCLAIMER

The information provided in this book, is for educational and informational purposes only and is not intended as medical advice. The content is not a substitute for professional medical advice, diagnosis, or treatment. Always seek the advice of your physician or other qualified health provider with any questions you may have regarding a medical condition. Never disregard professional medical advice or delay in seeking it because of something you have read in this book.

The dietary suggestions and recipes in this book are based on general guidelines and may not be suitable for everyone. Individual responses to foods can vary, and it is important to consult with a healthcare professional before making any significant changes to your diet.

The author and publisher of this book do not claim to cure or treat any medical condition. The information provided is based on research and personal experience and is intended to help readers make informed decisions about their diet and health.

Furthermore, I the author do not endorse any specific products, brands, treatments, or services that may be mentioned in this book. Any references to products, services, websites, or organizations are provided for informational purposes only and do not constitute an endorsement or recommendation by the author. The inclusion of such references does not imply any association, sponsorship, or affiliation between the author and the referenced entities.

The recipes and dietary suggestions in this book are designed to be safe and healthful. However, readers should use their own discretion and consult with a healthcare professional when necessary, especially if they have allergies, sensitivities, or other dietary restrictions.

By using this book, you acknowledge and agree that the author and publisher shall not be held liable for any loss or damage, including but not limited to special, incidental, consequential, or other damages, resulting from the use of the information and recipes contained in this book.

ABOUT THIS BOOK

This "EXOCRINE PANCREATIC INSUFFICIENCY (EPI) DIET COOKBOOK" is an essential resource for individuals who are impacted by EPI. It offers a comprehensive aid to the understanding, management, and daily living of this difficult condition. This book commences with a perceptive description of the causes and symptoms of Exocrine Pancreatic Insufficiency, as well as the critical role that the pancreas performs indigestion. The text emphasizes the substantial influence that dietary modifications can have on an individual's digestive health and overall well-being, thereby recognizing the significance of a customized diet in the management of EPI.

To comprehend EPI, it is necessary to identify the symptoms and endure the requisite diagnostic procedures to guarantee effective management.

This book delves into the critical function of the pancreas in digestion, emphasizing the impact of EPI on nutrient absorption and the resulting numerous digestive challenges. It also explores the potential long-term health consequences of untreated EPI and provides a comprehensive overview of the standard treatment options that are available to patients.

It is impossible to exaggerate the significance of diet in the management of EPI. This cookbook delineates the impact of particular dietary choices on digestive health, with a particular emphasis on the unique challenges that individuals with EPI encounter in terms of nutrient assimilation. Patients can enhance their quality of life and more effectively manage their symptoms by adhering to essential dietary principles and incorporating enzyme replacement therapy. Additionally, This book discusses the significance of essential vitamins and supplements in guaranteeing sufficient nutrition.

Individuals with EPI require diets that are abundant in nutrients. Detailed guidance on essential nutrients is provided in this book, which recommends foods that are abundant in essential vitamins and minerals, which are essential for maintaining digestive health. It underscores the significance of incorporating fruits and vegetables, high-protein foods, and healthful lipids into one's diet. Furthermore, the significance of fiber and the importance of adequate hydration is extensively examined to facilitate the effective management of EPI symptoms.

This cookbook emphasizes the importance of developing a diet plan that is customized to the requirements of EPI. It provides detailed instructions for creating nutritious meal plans, including sample menus and practical advice for meal preparation. The significance of portion control and the necessity of adapting meal plans to meet the unique requirements of each individual are underscored, thereby guaranteeing that dietary management is both effective and personalized.

Comprehensively addressed are common concerns associated with EPI, including managing weight loss, managing digestive distress, and navigating social situations. This book serves as a practical guide for real-life scenarios by offering strategies for managing social gatherings, dining out, and traveling with EPI. Additionally, responses to frequently requested concerns are provided, providing readers with a sense of assurance and clarity.

Specifically advantageous are the chapters that specialize in meal planning and preparation. They consist of sample meal plans that are tailored to meet the caloric requirements of various individuals, advice on bulk preparation, and the significance of meal timing and frequency. Practical advice and innovative suggestions facilitate the adaptation of recipes to be EPI-friendly.

This cookbook's compilation of nutritious and delectable recipes that are specifically designed for individuals with EPI is a standout feature. It includes a diverse selection of recipes for breakfast, lunch, dinner, snacking, and desserts, all of which are intended to be both satiating and by the dietary guidelines of the EPI.

These recipes are not only nutritious but also pleasurable, which enhances the experience of adhering to a diet.

Social situations and dining out can be difficult for individuals with EPI; however, this book offers valuable advice on how to effectively communicate dietary requirements, manage social gatherings, and dine out. It provides strategies for locating EPI-friendly options at restaurants and preparing for travel, thereby guaranteeing that social activities are stress-free and pleasurable.

More than just diet is required to maintain a healthy lifestyle with EPI. The significance of maintaining an active lifestyle, managing stress, and receiving routine medical examinations is emphasized in this book, as they all have an impact on digestive health. To achieve long-term administration and well-being, it is essential to establish a support system and consistently monitor and modify one's diet. This cookbook is not merely a dietary guide; it is a comprehensive manual for leading a more balanced and healthier existence with EPI.

CHAPTER ONE

Comprehending Exocrine Pancreatic Insufficiency (EPI)

Exocrine Pancreatic Insufficiency (EPI) is a condition in which the pancreas is unable to generate an adequate quantity of digestive enzymes to facilitate the digestion of food. Malabsorption and nutritional deficiencies result from the body's inability to break down lipids, proteins, and carbohydrates in the absence of these enzymes.

Definition And Causes Of EPI

Chronic pancreatitis, cystic fibrosis, pancreatic cancer, and specific gastrointestinal procedures are among the numerous factors that can induce EPI. Furthermore, EPI may be exacerbated by conditions such as diabetes and autoimmune disorders. EPI can be the result of any condition that impairs the pancreas's function or damages it.

Symptoms And Diagnosis

The symptoms of EPI may include excessive flatulence, bloating, abdominal discomfort, diarrhea, and weight loss. To evaluate the structure and function of the pancreas, a combination of medical history, physical examination, and tests such as fecal elastase or stool lipid tests, blood tests, and imaging studies like CT scans or MRIs is typically employed in the diagnosis.

The Function Of The Pancreas In Digestion

The pancreas is essential for metabolism as it produces digestive enzymes, such as amylase, lipase, and proteases, which aid in the digestion of carbohydrates, lipids, and proteins, respective, respectively. These enzymes are released into the small intestine, where they facilitate the digestion and absorption of nutrients from food.

The Significance Of Diet In The Management Of EPI

Diet is essential for the effective management of EPI symptoms and the correct absorption of nutrients. A personalized dietary plan that is customized to the unique requirements of an individual can be developed with the assistance of a dietitian.

In general, individuals with EPI may benefit from a low-fat diet that emphasizes readily digestible foods, such as lean proteins, fruits, vegetables, and whole grains. Symptoms such as diarrhea and abdominal discomfort can be alleviated by refraining from consuming high-fat and oily foods.

Treatment Options Overview

The primary objectives of EPI treatment are to alleviate symptoms, enhance nutrient absorption, and address the underlying cause. This frequently entails pancreatic enzyme replacement therapy (PERT), which entails the administration of digestive enzyme supplements with meals to facilitate digestion. Other treatments may involve the management of underlying conditions, lifestyle changes, dietary modifications, and, in severe cases, surgery. To effectively manage EPI and maintain overall health, it may be necessary to make regular adjustments to treatment plans and monitor the condition.

Diet In The Management Of EPI

Exocrine Pancreatic Insufficiency (EPI) is effectively managed through the implementation of a meticulously designed diet. The appropriate diet can alleviate symptoms and enhance overall health, as EPI impairs the pancreas' capacity to produce digestive enzymes. Individuals with EPI can substantially improve their quality of life by selecting foods that are both easily digestible and abundant in essential nutrients.

Digestive Health and Diet: The foods we consume have a direct impact on digestive health, particularly for individuals with EPI. Certain foods may exacerbate symptoms such as diarrhea, flatulence, and bloating, while others can facilitate digestion and enhance nutrient absorption. For example, individuals with EPI may experience distress and malabsorption as a result of the difficulty of digesting high-fat and high-fiber foods.

Nutrient Absorption Challenges in EPI: The insufficient production of pancreatic enzymes in EPI presents significant challenges to nutrient absorption. Malnutrition and deficiencies result from the body's inability to digest lipids, proteins, and carbohydrates in the absence of sufficient enzymes. This emphasizes the necessity of implementing a diet that addresses these deficiencies and guarantees an adequate intake of nutrients.

Benefits of a Well-Planned Diet: A diet that is specifically designed for individuals with EPI can provide a variety of advantages, such as enhanced digestion, reduced gastrointestinal symptoms, and improved nutrient assimilation.

Individuals with EPI can improve their overall health and quality of life by emphasizing readily digestible foods and optimizing their nutrient intake. For instance, symptoms can be effectively managed by avoiding trigger foods and consuming smaller, more frequent meals.

Enzyme replacement therapy (ERT) is a fundamental component of the administration of EPI. These enzyme supplements assist in compensating for the absence of pancreatic enzymes, thereby facilitating the correct assimilation of nutrients and digestion.

ERT can considerably alleviate symptoms and prevent complications associated with EPI when used in conjunction with a suitable diet, enabling individuals to lead more comfortable and fulfilling lives.

CHAPTER TWO

EPI-Friendly Nutrient-Rich Foods

It is essential to concentrate on foods that are high in nutrients when managing Exocrine Pancreatic Insufficiency (EPI). Choose lean proteins, such as tofu, fish, and chicken, as they are more easily digestible and contain essential amino acids.

To facilitate the assimilation of nutrients, incorporate healthful lipids from sources such as avocados, nuts, and olive oil. Incorporate complex carbohydrates, including whole cereals, fruits, and vegetables, which are essential for maintaining overall health by providing fiber, vitamins, and minerals.

Dairy products, such as yogurt and cheese, can also be advantageous; however, individuals with lactose intolerance should opt for lactose-free alternatives.

Essential Nutrients For Digestive Health

Maintaining an adequate consumption of essential nutrients is of the utmost importance for individuals with EPI. Malabsorption may result in a deficiency of fat-soluble vitamins A, D, E, and K, which are critical nutrients.

To satisfy these requirements, contemplate the consumption of fortified foods or supplementation. Furthermore, prioritize the acquisition of an adequate amount of calcium and magnesium to maintain enzyme function and bone health.

Omega-3 fatty acids, which are present in flaxseeds and fish, can be beneficial for gastrointestinal health and inflammation reduction.

Foods That Should Be Incorporated Into An EPI Diet

Selecting foods that are both nutrient-dense and readily digestible is a critical component of constructing an EPI-friendly diet. Choose cooked vegetables over fresh ones, as they are less taxing on the digestive system. Select protein sources that are low in cholesterol, such as poultry, fish, and plant-based options like lentils and legumes. To facilitate digestion and prevent the pancreas from becoming overburdened, consume small, frequent meals throughout the day.

Incorporate carbohydrates that are readily digestible, such as rice, quinoa, and cereals, to ensure that the digestive system is not overtaxed and that sustained energy is provided.

Foods To Avoid

Certain substances can exacerbate symptoms of EPI and should be avoided or restricted.

High-fat foods, such as fried items, fatty cuts of meat, and creamy condiments, can be uncomfortable and overtax the compromised digestive system. It is advisable to limit the consumption of fresh vegetables and fruits with firm skins or seeds, as they may be difficult to metabolize. Reduce or eliminate the consumption of dairy products that are high in lactose, and instead choose lactose-free alternatives. In addition, it is advisable to restrict the consumption of processed foods that contain artificial ingredients and added carbohydrates, as they provide minimal nutritional value and may exacerbate gastrointestinal distress.

The Function Of Fiber In The Management Of EPI

Although fiber is crucial for digestive health, individuals with EPI may need to exercise caution when consuming it.

Insoluble fiber, which is present in foods such as whole cereals and specific vegetables, can be difficult to digest and may exacerbate symptoms. Alternatively, concentrate on soluble fiber sources such as vegetables, pears, and oats, which are less abrasive on the digestive system.

It is essential to maintain adequate hydration when increasing fiber intake, as it aids in the prevention of constipation and the promotion of regular bowel movements.

The Significance Of Hydration

Individuals with EPI require adequate hydration to facilitate digestion and promote overall health. It is recommended that you consume an abundance of water throughout the day, particularly during meals, to facilitate the assimilation and digestion of nutrients.

In addition to alleviating digestive discomfort, herbal teas, and clear broths can also contribute to fluid intake.

Refrain from consuming caffeinated and alcoholic beverages in excess, as they can exacerbate EPI symptoms and contribute to dehydration. Ensuring that urine color and frequency are monitored can assist in the preservation of sufficient hydration levels.

CHAPTER THREE

Formulating A Meal Plan For EPI

Focus on foods that are low in fat and simple to metabolize when developing a meal plan for Exocrine Pancreatic Insufficiency (EPI). Begin by incorporating carbohydrates, such as rice, potatoes, and pasta, and lean proteins, such as chicken, fish, and tofu.

Consume an abundance of fruits and vegetables, preferring prepared or canned varieties over fresh ones to facilitate digestion. Restrict the consumption of high-fat foods, such as fatty meats, decadent sauces, and sautéed dishes, as they may exacerbate symptoms. To alleviate the burden on the digestive system, strive for smaller, more frequent meals throughout the day. Consult with a registered dietitian to develop a plan that is customized to your requirements.

Methods For Formulating A Well-Balanced Meal Plan

To begin, ascertain your calorie requirements by considering factors such as age, weight, activity level, and metabolic rate. Subsequently, allocate your daily caloric intake among macronutrients in equitable proportions: carbohydrates, proteins, and lipids.

To guarantee that your body's requirements are satisfied, strive to consume a diverse array of nutrient-dense foods. Incorporate fiber-rich foods, such as whole cereals, fruits, and vegetables, to promote digestive health.

Avoid excessive servings and be mindful of portion sizes, as they can result in digestive issues and discomfort. Finally, pay attention to your body's signals and modify your meal plan accordingly.

Meal Plans Examples

A typical day's meal plan for an individual with EPI may consist of a breakfast of oatmeal with banana slices and almond butter, a mid-morning snack of Greek yogurt with honey, a lunch of grilled chicken breast with quinoa and steamed vegetables, an afternoon snack of apple slices with peanut butter, and a dinner of baked salmon with sweet potato and spinach. To maintain hydration and facilitate digestion, it is important to consume an ample amount of water throughout the day.

Strategies For Meal Preparation

Meal preparation can facilitate the EPI diet by guaranteeing that you have nutritious meals readily available, particularly during periods of high activity. Each week, allocate a day to the planning and preparation of your meals. Select recipes that are simple to prepare in large quantities and can be divided into portions for multiple meals. To maintain the freshness of your meals, allocate funds toward high-quality storage containers. It is advisable to pre-cut vegetables and ration out munchies for on-the-go consumption. To maintain the freshness of your food and ensure that older dishes are rotated to the front of the fridge, label your containers with the date.

Significance Of Portion Control

Portion control is essential for the management of EPI symptoms, as the digestive system can be overburdened and discomfort may result. Utilize balances and measuring containers to accurately measure out the appropriate portion sizes of foods.

Be aware of the size of restaurant portions, as they are frequently excessively enormous.

Attempt to occupy half of your plate with non-starchy vegetables, a quarter with lean protein, and a quarter with whole cereals or starchy vegetables. Additionally, digestion can be facilitated and overeating can be avoided by consuming slowly and digesting food thoroughly. Adapt the quantity of the portions to suit your personal preferences and requirements.

Frequently Asked Questions And Common Concerns

Common concerns for individuals with EPI frequently pertain to comprehension of the condition, its symptoms, and management strategies.

FAQs may encompass inquiries regarding lifestyle modifications, enzyme replacement therapy, and dietary restrictions.

It is imperative to address these concerns with precise information and offer assurance regarding the effective management of EPI.

Weight loss management with EPI: The optimization of enzyme replacement therapy and the consumption of nutrient-dense foods that are easily digestible are the primary components of weight loss management with EPI.

The consumption of modest, frequent meals that are high in proteins, healthful fats, and carbohydrates can aid in the maintenance or gain of weight. Identifying catalysts for weight loss and modifying the diet accordingly can also be facilitated by monitoring food intake and symptoms. Personalized guidance and support can be obtained by consulting with a dietitian who is proficient in EPI management.

Managing digestive discomfort: Digestion is a frequent obstacle for individuals with EPI, frequently presenting as diarrhea, abdominal pain, flatulence, and bloating. It is essential to steer clear of trigger foods, such as high-fat or high-fiber items, to alleviate these symptoms. Instead, it is recommended to prioritize readily digestible options, such as lean proteins, cooked vegetables, and refined cereals. Furthermore, the administration of digestive enzymes in the prescribed dosage can facilitate the digestion of food and alleviate discomfort. Maintaining a food diary can assist in the identification of specific triggers and the subsequent adjustment of the diet.

Traveling with EPI necessitates meticulous preparation to guarantee that the patient has access to the necessary medications and consumables while away from home. It is imperative to bring a sufficient quantity of digestive enzymes, as well as refreshments that are readily transportable, such as protein bars, nuts, and seeds.

Conducting preliminary research on the restaurant options available at the destination can assist in the identification of EPI-friendly options and the avoidance of potential triggers. In the event of any travel-related issues, it is also recommended to travel with a letter from a healthcare provider that elucidates the necessity of enzyme replacement therapy.

Eating out and social situations: While navigating social situations with EPI can be challenging, it is feasible with adequate preparation and communication. Selecting restaurants that offer customizable or easily digestible options, such as grilled meats, steamed vegetables, and simple carbohydrates, can assist in alleviating symptoms when dining out. Ensuring that dishes are prepared to meet EPI requirements can be achieved by communicating dietary demands to servers or chefs.

Furthermore, the provision of digestive enzymes and refreshments can offer reassurance if there are insufficient suitable options. Fostering understanding and support in social contexts can also be achieved by engaging in frank dialogue with friends and family about dietary restrictions.

Answers to frequently asked questions: Dietary choices, enzyme replacement therapy, and lifestyle adjustments are frequently the subjects of frequently asked questions about EPI. Empowering individuals to effectively manage their condition and alleviate concerns can be achieved by providing plain and concise responses that are supported by evidence. Providing individuals with EPI with resources such as educational materials, support groups, and reputable websites can further assist them in navigating life.

CHAPTER FOUR

Foods To Avoid And The Reasons For Their Avoidance

To effectively manage EPI, it is essential to avoid high-fat foods, as they can exacerbate symptoms as a result of the pancreas' inability to generate an adequate amount of digestive enzymes. Foods such as sautéed foods, creamy sauces, fatty types of meat, and full-fat dairy products should be strictly avoided, as they may induce symptoms such as abdominal pain, bloating, and diarrhea. Instead, choose lean proteins, low-fat dairy, and healthful lipids such as nuts and avocados.

Foods That Exacerbate Symptoms Of EPI

EPI symptoms can be exacerbated by specific foods, which can further complicate digestion. These foods, such as legumes, whole cereals, and cruciferous vegetables, are high in fiber and may be challenging to digest in the absence of adequate enzymes. Furthermore, the digestive system may be irritated and symptoms may be exacerbated by piquant foods, caffeine, and alcohol. By choosing smaller, more frequent meals and refraining from these trigger foods, it is possible to alleviate discomfort.

Comprehending Trigger Ingredients

It is imperative to comprehend trigger foods to effectively manage EPI symptoms. Frequent triggers include caffeine, alcohol, high-fat foods, and piquant foods, although the specific foods can differ from person to person.

Maintaining a food diary can assist in the identification of specific trigger foods and facilitate the more effective management of symptoms. Valuable insight into personal triggers can be gained by experimenting with various foods and observing their impact on digestion.

Substitutes For Prevalently Problematic Cuisines

It is crucial to identify appropriate substitutes for common problematic foods to maintain a balanced diet and reduce symptoms when confronted with EPI. For instance, instead of consuming high-fat dairy products such as whole milk, consider lactose-free or low-fat alternatives. Opt for roasted or grilled alternatives instead of fried dishes.

Additionally, it may be advantageous to incorporate additional plant-based proteins, such as legumes and tofu. These alternatives supply nutrients without overtaxing the digestive system.

Comprehending And Interpreting Food Labels

Individuals with EPI need to read and comprehend food labels to prevent the consumption of constituents that may provoke symptoms. Search for terms such as "high-fat," "fried," or "creamy" on food labels, as they represent foods that may exacerbate symptoms. Furthermore, it is important to be cautious of the presence of carbohydrates and lipids that are concealed in processed foods.

To reduce the likelihood of symptom flare-ups, select products that are labeled as "reduced sugar," "lean," or "low-fat." It is also beneficial to become acquainted with the effects of common food additives to make more informed decisions at the grocery store.

Meal Planning And Preparation

Meal planning for individuals with exocrine pancreatic insufficiency (EPI) entails the preparation of nutritious, well-balanced meals that are easily digestible. Begin by emphasizing smaller, more frequent meals throughout the day to facilitate digestion. Combine a diverse array of carbohydrates, including rice, potatoes, and cereals, with protein sources such as lean meats, fish, tofu, and eggs. Incorporate nutritious lipids from sources such as avocado, almonds, and olive oil. Opt for culinary methods such as baking, steaming, or grilling instead of frying, and steer clear of high-fat, oily foods.

Methods For Formulating An Efficient Diet Schedule

To begin, ascertain your daily caloric requirements by considering factors such as age, gender, weight, and activity level. To facilitate improved digestion and assimilation, distribute these calories among smaller meals and nibbles throughout the day. Plan meals that are well-balanced in terms of protein, carbohydrates, and lipids to guarantee that you receive the necessary nutrients. Consult with a dietitian to develop a nutrition plan that is customized to your unique requirements and preferences.

Sample Menu Arrangements For Varying Caloric Requirements

Sample meal plans can offer advice on food selections and portion sizes for individuals with diverse caloric requirements.

For instance, a 1500-calorie meal plan could encompass a variety of options, such as oatmeal with fruit and almonds for breakfast, a turkey and avocado wrap with a side salad for lunch, grilled chicken with quinoa and roasted vegetables for dinner, and Greek yogurt with blueberries for a refreshment. For individuals with calorie requirements that are either higher or lower, adjust their portion sizes and food selections accordingly.

Recommendations For Recipe Preparation And Batch Cooking

Batch preparation and meal preparation can ensure that you have EPI-friendly meals readily available, while also saving time and energy. Select recipes that are readily scalable and can be preserved for future use.

Invest in high-quality storage containers to divide out meals in advance, facilitating the process of grabbing and going when necessary. Cooking substantial quantities of proteins, cereals, and vegetables at the commencement of the week can facilitate the creation of a variety of meals.

The Significance Of Feeding Timing And Frequency

It is imperative to maintain consistent meal timing and frequency to optimize nutrient absorption and manage EPI symptoms.

Aim to consume food every 3-4 hours to prevent the digestive system from becoming overloaded and to maintain consistent energy levels. It is advisable to refrain from avoiding meals or going for extended periods without consuming, as this can exacerbate symptoms and result in nutritional deficiencies.

To ascertain the appropriate timing and quantity of each meal and refreshment, pay attention to your body's appetite and fullness signals.

CHAPTER FIVE

Recipes That Are Both Nutritious And Delicious

It is essential to maintain a diet that is both nutritious and delectable to effectively manage Exocrine Pancreatic Insufficiency (EPI). Select recipes that are abundant in essential nutrients and contain ingredients that are easily digestible. Pair complex carbohydrates, such as sweet potatoes, quinoa, and brown rice, with lean proteins, such as skinless poultry, fish, and tofu. Increase your vitamin and mineral intake by consuming a variety of vibrant fruits and vegetables.

Experiment with herbs and seasonings to improve the flavor without introducing additional oil or sodium.

Breakfast Recipes: Simple And Rapid Alternatives

Begin your day with breakfast options that are both nutritious and easy on the digestive system. For an additional source of protein and beneficial lipids, consider a smoothie that contains spinach, banana, low-fat yogurt, and a spoonful of almond butter. Alternatively, savor a dish of oatmeal with cut strawberries and a drizzle of honey. If you prefer a savory dish, prepare scrambled eggs with minced vegetables such as spinach, mushrooms, and bell peppers.

Lunch Recipes: Nutritious And Satisfying Meals

Aim for balanced meals that offer sustained energy and contentment for lunch. Create a vegetarian quinoa salad that includes grilled chicken or chickpeas, cucumber, cherry tomatoes, and avocado. Drizzle with a mild vinaigrette that is composed of lemon juice, olive oil, and seasonings. An additional alternative is a whole-grain tortilla that is stuffed with grilled vegetables, hummus, and cubed turkey or tofu. For an additional source of fiber and vitamins, accompany the dish with a small serving of citrus and a side of uncooked vegetables.

Dinner Recipes: Delicious And Well-Received Meals

Develop delectable entrees that are customized to your dietary requirements and taste preferences. Opt for steamed or roasted vegetables, such as broccoli, carrots, and cauliflower, to accompany broiled or grilled proteins, such as salmon, chicken, or lean cuts of beef. As a nutritious side dish, prepare quinoa pilaf that is seasoned with garlic, shallot, and seasonings. Opt for light marinades or dressings that are composed of ingredients such as honey, balsamic vinegar, and Dijon mustard, rather than heavier sauces or fried dishes.

Healthy And Satisfying Snack Recipes

Keep appetite at bay between meals by consuming nutritious and gratifying snacks. A balanced combination of protein, healthy lipids, and fiber can be achieved by consuming a fistful of almonds or walnuts in conjunction with a piece of fruit.

A nutritious refreshment that is both calcium-rich and probiotic-rich is achieved by topping Greek yogurt with cherries and a sprinkling of granola. Veggie skewers with hummus or a small serving of whole-grain crackers with cottage cheese are also excellent choices for maintaining energy levels throughout the day.

Dessert Recipes: Indulgent And EPI-Friendly Desserts

Indulge your sugar tooth with delicacies that are both indulgent and appropriate for managing EPI. Use pureed banana or applesauce as a natural sweetener in place of sugar when baking several oatmeal cookies.

Add moisture and nutrients to pastries or cakes by incorporating grated zucchini or carrots. For a velvety texture without lactose, consider using dairy-free alternatives such as almond milk or coconut milk in pudding or custard recipes.

It is important to remember to consume desserts in moderation and to be mindful of portion sizes to maintain a healthy diet.

CHAPTER SIX

Eating Out And Handling Social Situations

It is imperative to organize one's culinary experience with EPI in advance. Seek out restaurants that provide EPI-friendly options, including plain rice or potatoes, steamed vegetables, and grilled or roasted lean proteins. Ensure that your meal is prepared without high-fat ingredients or excessive oils by explicitly communicating your dietary needs to the waiter or chef. Steer clear of fried foods, creamy sauces, and dishes that contain excessive amounts of butter or cheese.

To prevent digestive issues or discomfort, it is advisable to consume smaller, more frequent meals. Do not hesitate to inquire about the preparation of a menu item if you are uncertain.

When dining out with EPI, it is beneficial to conduct preliminary research on restaurants and select those that accommodate your dietary requirements. Look for dishes that are simple to digest and low in cholesterol, such as grilled chicken or fish with steamed vegetables. Steer clear of fried foods, hefty condiments, and dishes that are high in dairy or butter. Consider requesting menu modifications, such as substituting basic, steamed side dishes for sauces on the side. Ensure that your meal is prepared according to your dietary demands by explicitly communicating them to the waiter or chef.

How To Manage Social Gatherings And Parties

While it may be difficult to navigate social gatherings and parties with EPI, it is feasible with adequate preparation. It is advisable to consume a modest, low-fat supper before attending an event to prevent hunger and discomfort at a later time. Inquire with the host or organizer about the availability of EPI-friendly options and inform them of your dietary restrictions. If feasible, please bring a dish that is compatible with your dietary requirements to contribute. Avoid overindulging or exacerbating digestive symptoms by engaging in social activities rather than solely focusing on food during the event. Additionally, it is important to regulate oneself when consuming.

Effectively communicating one's dietary requirements is essential for the management of EPI. Do not hesitate to disclose your condition and specific dietary restrictions to stewards, chefs, or hostesses when dining out or attending social occasions. Make it clear which foods you must avoid and any necessary modifications to your meals. This information can assist others in comprehending the significance of accommodating your dietary requirements by providing information about EPI and its effect on digestion. Advocating for oneself should be conducted in a manner that is both assertive and courteous. Do not hesitate to ask inquiries or make requests to guarantee one's safety and well-being.

Finding EPI-Friendly Restaurant Options

It is imperative to select restaurants that provide appropriate menu options when dining out with EPI. Seek out restaurants that prioritize the use of fresh, whole ingredients and provide the option to customize their dishes.

Select lean proteins, such as grilled chicken or fish, and side dishes, such as simple rice or steamed vegetables. Refrain from consuming dishes that contain hefty condiments, excessive oils, or fried preparations. Some restaurants may even have designated EPI-friendly sections on their menus or be willing to accommodate special requests.

Please do not hesitate to ask about the ingredients or preparation methods to guarantee that your dish meets your dietary requirements.

CHAPTER SEVEN

Seven-Day Meal Plan, Ingredients, And Detailed Preparatory Guidelines For Exocrine Pancreatic Insufficiency

DAY ONE:

Breakfast: Banana Oatmeal Smoothie

- **INGREDIENTS**:

o One mature banana

o ½ cup of dried oats

o One cup of almond milk (or any other non-dairy milk)

o One tablespoon of honey (optional)

- ***DIRECTIONS:***

1. All ingredients should be blended until they are homogeneous.

2. Chill before serving.

Quinoa Salad for Lunch

- **INGREDIENTS**:

o One cup of prepared quinoa

o One cup of minced cucumber

o One cup of cherry tomatoes, halved

o One-half cup of roasted legumes

o Two tablespoons of olive oil

o One tablespoon of lemon juice

o Add salt and pepper to taste

• **DIRECTIONS:**

1. Quinoa, cucumber, tomatoes, and chickpeas should be combined in a sizable basin.

2. Drizzle lemon juice and olive oil over the salad.

3. Sprinkle salt and pepper over the dish, mix thoroughly, and serve.

Dinner: Steamed Vegetables with Baked Salmon

• **INGREDIENTS:**

o Two salmon fillets

o One lemon, cut

2 cups of a variety of vegetables, including broccoli, carrots, and zucchini

o Two tablespoons of olive oil

o Add salt and pepper to taste

- **DIRECTIONS:**

1. Preheat the oven to 375°F (190°C).

2. Arrange the salmon fillets on a baking sheet that has been lined with parchment paper.

3. Place lemon segments on top of the salmon, drizzle with olive oil, and season with salt and pepper.

4. Bake the salmon for 15-20 minutes or until it is fully cooked.

5. In the interim, steam the assorted vegetables until they are soft.

6. Steamed vegetables should accompany the broiled salmon.

Snack: Honey-dipped Greek Yogurt

- **INGREDIENTS:**

o One cup of Greek yogurt

o One tablespoon of honey

• DIRECTIONS:

1. Honey and Greek yogurt should be combined in a basin.

2. Combine thoroughly and relish as a refreshment.

DAY TWO:

Breakfast: Scrambled Eggs with Spinach

• INGREDIENTS:

o Two eggs

o One cup of freshly minced spinach

o One tablespoon of olive oil

• DIRECTIONS:

1. Heat olive oil in a pan over medium heat.

2. Add spinach and simmer until it is wilted.

3. Scramble the eggs in the pan until they are fully cooked.

4. Serve at a high temperature.

Lunch: Lentil Soup

- **INGREDIENTS**:

o One cup of drained dried legumes

o One diced onion

o Two carrots, cut

o Two minced celery stalks

o Four pints of vegetable broth

o One teaspoon of dried thyme

o Add salt and pepper to taste

- **DIRECTIONS:**

1. Sauté celery, carrots, and onion in a substantial saucepan until they are tender.

2. Incorporate dried thyme, vegetable bouillon, and lentils.

3. Bring the mixture to a boil, then reduce the heat and allow it to simmer for 20-25 minutes, or until the lentils are tender.

4. Before serving, add salt and pepper.

Dinner: Stir-fried turkey and Vegetables

- **INGREDIENTS**:

o One pound of thinly cut turkey breast

o Two cups of a variety of vegetables, including mushrooms, snap peas, and bell peppers

o Two teaspoons of soy sauce

o One tablespoon of olive oil

o One teaspoon of minced garlic

• ***DIRECTIONS:***

1. Heat olive oil in a large pan or wok over medium-high heat.

2. Add minced garlic and sliced turkey breast to the pan; sauté until the poultry is browned.

3. Add soy sauce and a mixture of vegetables; stir-fry until the vegetables are soft.

4. Serve at a high temperature.

Snack: Apple slices with almond butter

• **INGREDIENTS**:

o One apple, cut

o Two tablespoons of almond butter

• *DIRECTIONS:*

1. Apply almond butter to apple segments.

2. Enjoy as a nutritious nibble.

THIRD DAY:

Breakfast: Chia Pudding with Blueberries

• **INGREDIENTS**:

o One-half cup of chia seeds

o 1 ½ glasses of almond milk (or any other non-dairy milk)

o One cup of blueberries

o One tablespoon of maple syrup (optional)

• *DIRECTIONS:*

1. Combine almond milk and chia seeds in a basin.

2. Incorporate maple syrup and blueberries.

3. The pudding should be refrigerated for a minimum of 2 hours or overnight until it thickens.

4. Chill before serving.

Lunch: Grilled Chicken Salad

• INGREDIENTS:

o Two boneless, skinless poultry breasts

o Four quarts of assorted greens

o One cup of cherry tomatoes, halved

o One-half cup of cut cucumber

o One-quarter cup of balsamic vinaigrette

• *DIRECTIONS:*

1. Sprinkle salt and pepper over poultry breasts.

2. Grill the chicken until it is fully cooked, and then divide it.

3. Cherry tomatoes, cucumber, and assorted greens should be combined in a sizable basin.

4. Drizzle balsamic vinaigrette over the sliced chicken.

5. Mix thoroughly and serve.

Dinner: Roasted Vegetables with Baked Cod

- **INGREDIENTS**:

o Two cod fillets

o Two tablespoons of olive oil

o One teaspoon of dried oregano

o One teaspoon of minced garlic

o Add salt and pepper to taste

o Two cups of a variety of vegetables, including zucchini, shallots, and bell peppers

- **DIRECTIONS:**

1. Set oven temperature to 400°F, or 200°C.

2. Combine olive oil, minced garlic, dried oregano, salt, and pepper in a basin.

3. Line a baking sheet with parchment paper and place the cod fillets on it.

4. Apply the olive oil mixture to the cod fillets.

5. Arrange a variety of vegetables around the cod.

6. Bake for 15-20 minutes or until the vegetables are tender and the cod is fully cooked.

7. Serve at a high temperature.

Snack: Hummus with Carrot Sticks

- **INGREDIENTS**:

2 carrots, cut into pieces

o One-third cup of hummus

- *DIRECTIONS:*

1. Serve carrot spears with hummus as a nutritious appetizer.

DAY FOUR:

Avocado Toast for Breakfast

- **INGREDIENTS**:

o Two slices of buttered whole-grain bread

o One mature avocado

o One teaspoon of lemon juice

o Add salt and pepper to taste

- **DIRECTIONS:**

1. Lemon juice, salt, and pepper are combined to mash the avocado.

2. Spread pureed avocado on slices of toasted bread.

3. Serve immediately.

Lunch: Quinoa Bowl with Vegetables

- **INGREDIENTS:**

o One cup of prepared quinoa

o One cup of roasted sweet potatoes

o One cup of sautéed kale

o 1/2 cup of black beans that have been simmered

o Two tablespoons of tahini vinaigrette

• DIRECTIONS:

1. Layer cooked quinoa, sautéed kale, roasted sweet potatoes, and black beans in a bowl.

2. Apply a tahini condiment to the dish.

3. Mix thoroughly and serve.

Dinner: Turkey Meatballs with Zucchini Noodles

• INGREDIENTS:

o One pound of minced poultry

o One egg

o One-third cup of breadcrumbs

o One teaspoon of Italian seasoning

o Add salt and pepper to taste

o Two spiralized zucchinis

o One cup of marinara sauce

- **DIRECTIONS:**

1. Preheat the oven to 375°F (190°C).

2. Combine minced turkey, egg, breadcrumbs, Italian seasoning, salt, and pepper in a basin.

3. Form the mixture into meatballs and arrange them on a baking sheet that has been lined with parchment paper.

4. Bake the meatballs for 20-25 minutes or until they are fully cooked.

5. In the interim, sauté spiralized zucchini in a pan until they are tender.

6. Serve turkey meatballs with marinara sauce and zucchini linguine.

Snack: Rice Cake with Peanut Butter

- **INGREDIENTS**:

o One rice cake

o One tablespoon of peanut butter

- *DIRECTIONS:*

1. Apply peanut butter to the rice cake.

2. Enjoy as a crispy nibble.

DAY FIVE:

Breakfast: Greek Yogurt Parfait

- **INGREDIENTS**:

o One cup of Greek yogurt

o 1/2 cup of granola

one-half cup of assorted fruit

- *DIRECTIONS*:

1. Layer Greek yogurt, granola, and assorted berries in a glass.

2. Continue the process of layering.

3. Chill before serving.

Lunch: Tuna Salad Lettuce Wraps

- **INGREDIENTS**:

  o One tuna can, drained

  o Two tablespoons of Greek yogurt

  o One tablespoon of lemon juice

  o One celery stalk, minced

  o Add salt and pepper to taste

  o Four large lettuce fronds

- *DIRECTIONS:*

1. Combine tuna, Greek yogurt, lemon juice, diced celery, salt, and pepper in a basin.

2. Spoon tuna salad onto lettuce leaves.

3. Roll lettuce leaves into bundles.

4. Serve immediately.

Dinner: Baked Chicken with Steamed Asparagus

- **INGREDIENTS**:

o Two chicken breasts

o One tablespoon of olive oil

o One teaspoon of garlic powder

o Add salt and pepper to taste

o One pound of asparagus, trimmed

- ***DIRECTIONS:***

1. Preheat the oven to 400°F (200°C).

2. Rub chicken breasts with garlic powder, olive oil, salt, and pepper.

3. Arrange the chicken breasts on a baking sheet that has been lined with parchment paper.

4. Bake the chicken for 20-25 minutes or until it is fully cooked.

5. In the interim, steam asparagus until it is soft.

6. Steamed asparagus should be served alongside roasted poultry.

Snack: Cream cheese-covered celery sticks

- **INGREDIENTS**:

o Two celery stalks, divided into pieces

o Two teaspoons of cream cheese

- ***DIRECTIONS:***

1. Apply cream cheese to celery stalks.

2. Enjoy as a crispy nibble.

DAY SIX:

Breakfast: Berry Smoothie Bowl

• **INGREDIENTS**:

o One cup of a variety of berries, including raspberries, blueberries, and strawberries

o One banana, cut

o ½ cup of almond milk (or any other non-dairy milk)

o Two tablespoons of granola

• *DIRECTIONS:*

1. In a blender, incorporate almond milk, banana, and assorted berries.

2. Blend until the mixture is uniform.

3. Transfer to a receptacle and sprinkle with granola.

4. Serve immediately.

Lunch: Vegetable Soup

INGREDIENTS

o One diced onion

o Two carrots, cut

o Two minced celery stalks

o One diced potato

o Four pints of vegetable broth

o One teaspoon of dried thyme

o Add salt and pepper to taste

• ***DIRECTIONS:***

1. Sauté the onion, carrots, celery, and potato in a large saucepan until they are tender.

2. Incorporate dried thyme and vegetable bouillon.

3. Bring the mixture to a boil, then reduce the heat and allow it to simmer for 20-25 minutes, or until the vegetables are tender.

4. Before serving, add salt and pepper.

Dinner: Grilled Salmon with Roasted Vegetables

• **INGREDIENTS**:

o Two salmon fillets

o Two tablespoons of olive oil

o One teaspoon of lemon zest

o One teaspoon of minced garlic

o Add salt and pepper to taste

o Two cups of a variety of vegetables, including broccoli, scallions, and bell peppers

- **DIRECTIONS:**

1. Preheat the grill to medium-high temperature.

2. Combine olive oil, minced garlic, lemon zest, salt, and pepper in a basin.

3. Apply the olive oil mixture to the salmon fillets.

4. Grill the salmon for 4-5 minutes on each side or until it is fully cooked.

5. In the interim, combine the vegetables with the remaining olive oil mixture.

6. Roast vegetables in the oven at 400°F (200°C) for 15-20 minutes or until they are tender.

7. Serve roasted vegetables alongside broiled salmon.

Snack: Trail Mix

- **INGREDIENTS**:

o One-quarter cup of almonds

o Cashews, 1/4 cup

o Two teaspoons of dried currants

o Two tablespoons of dark chocolate chunks

- *DIRECTIONS:*

1. Combine all components.

2. Savor as a satisfying nibble.

SEVENTH DAY:

Breakfast: Omelet with Spinach and Mushrooms

- **INGREDIENTS**:

o Two eggs

o One cup of freshly minced spinach

o Sliced mushrooms, approximately ½ cup

o One tablespoon of olive oil

- ***DIRECTIONS:***

1. Heat olive oil in a pan over medium heat.

2. Incorporate spinach and mushrooms into the pan and simmer until they are tender.

3. In a basin, whisk the eggs and then pour the mixture over the spinach and mushrooms.

4. Cook the omelet until the eggs are fully cooked, and then divide it in half.

5. Serve at a high temperature.

Lunch: Stir-fry with Chicken and Vegetables

- **INGREDIENTS**:

o One pound of thinly cut chicken breast

o Two cups of a variety of vegetables, including carrots, snap peas, and bell peppers

o Two teaspoons of soy sauce

o One tablespoon of olive oil

o One teaspoon of minced garlic

- ***DIRECTIONS:***

1. Heat olive oil in a large pan or wok over medium-high heat.

2. Add sliced chicken breast and minced garlic; sauté until the chicken is browned.

3. Add soy sauce and a mixture of vegetables; stir-fry until the vegetables are soft.

4. Serve at a high temperature.

Vegetable and Bean Chili for Dinner

- **INGREDIENTS**:

  o One diced onion

  o Two minced garlic cloves

  o One minced bell pepper

  o One zucchini, minced

  o One can of diced tomatoes

  o One can of kidney beans, drained and rinsed

  o One tablespoon of chile powder

  o Add salt and pepper to taste

- *DIRECTIONS:*

1. Sauté zucchini, bell pepper, onion, and garlic in a sizable saucepan until they are tender.

2. Add minced tomatoes, kidney beans, chile powder, salt, and pepper.

3. Bring the mixture to a boil, then reduce the heat and allow it to simmer for 20-25 minutes.

4. Serve at a high temperature.

Snack: Pineapple and Cottage Cheese

- **INGREDIENTS**:

o One cup of cottage cheese

o 1/2 cup of fresh pineapple segments

- *DIRECTIONS*:

1. For a delightful nibble, combine pineapple slices with cottage cheese.

It is important to adjust the size of the portions and the ingredients to suit your dietary requirements and preferences. I hope you enjoy your meals!

CHAPTER EIGHT

7 Desserts Procedural Recipes For Exocrine Pancreatic Insufficiency (EPI) And Guidelines

Exocrine Pancreatic Insufficiency (EPI) is a condition in which the pancreas is unable to generate an adequate quantity of enzymes to correctly digest food, resulting in nutrient deficiencies and malabsorption. Dietary modifications, such as the consumption of readily digestible foods, moderate lipid intake, and the implementation of pancreatic enzyme replacement therapy, are essential for the management of EPI.

Desserts can be difficult to prepare due to their elevated sugar and calorie content. Nevertheless, it is feasible to create nutritious and pleasurable delicacies by meticulously selecting ingredients and implementing appropriate preparation techniques. Seven dessert recipes and guidelines that are EPI-friendly are provided to assist you in indulging in delectable delights without sacrificing your health.

1. BERRY YOGURT PARFAIT

INGREDIENTS:

• One cup of Greek yogurt (low-fat or fat-free)

• One cup of a combination of berries, including raspberries, blueberries, and strawberries

• One tablespoon of honey

• One teaspoon of vanilla extract

STEPS:

1. Combine honey and vanilla extract with Greek yogurt.

2. The yogurt mixture and berries are alternately layered in a glass until it is filled.

3. Let cool for half an hour before serving.

Guidelines: Greek yogurt is a source of probiotics and protein, which can help with digestion. Antioxidants and micronutrients are present in berries. Opt for low-fat versions to reduce the oil content, which will facilitate digestion.

2. APPLE CINNAMON BAKED SLICES

INGREDIENTS:

- Two large pears, sliced thinly

- One teaspoon of cinnamon

- One tablespoon of maple syrup

- One tablespoon of water

STEPS:

1. Preheat the oven to 350°F (175°C).

2. Arrange apple segments on a baking tray.

3. Combine water, maple syrup, and cinnamon, and apply the mixture to the fruits.

4. Until the fruits are tender, bake for 20-25 minutes.

Apples are abundant in vitamins and fiber. The fibers are softened by baking them, which facilitates digestion. Cinnamon enhances the flavor of food without introducing additional lipids.

3. CHIA SEED PUDDING

INGREDIENTS:

- One cup of strained almond milk

- Three tablespoons of chia seeds

- One tablespoon of honey

- One teaspoon of vanilla extract

STEPS:

1. Combine all ingredients in a dish.

2. Stir the mixture thoroughly to prevent the chia seeds from forming a cluster.

3. Allow the seeds to swell and develop a pudding-like texture by refrigerating them overnight.

Guidelines: Omega-3 fatty acids and fiber are abundant in chia seeds. Almond milk is lactose-free and low in cholesterol, rendering it an appropriate choice for patients with EPI.

4. MANGO SORBET

INGREDIENTS:

- Two mature mangoes, trimmed and cubed

- One tablespoon of citrus juice

- One tablespoon of honey

STEPS:

1. Mango segments should be blended until they are smooth.

2. Incorporate honey and citrus juice into the mixture and puree once more.

3. Stir occasionally to prevent the formation of ice crystals, and freeze for a minimum of four hours.

Mangoes are abundant in vitamins A and C. Sorbets are more easily digestible than traditional ice desserts due to their minimal fat content.

5. BANANA OAT COOKIES

INGREDIENTS:

- Two mature avocados

- One cup of rolled oats

- One teaspoon of cinnamon

- One teaspoonful of raisins (optional)

STEPS:

1. Set the oven's temperature to 175°C/350°F.

2. In a dish, mash bananas.

3. Mix in oats, cinnamon, and raisins, if desired.

4. Place spoonfuls of the mixture onto a baking sheet and gently press them down.

5. Bake for 15 minutes.

Guidelines: Bananas are a source of potassium and are naturally delicious. Additionally, oatmeal is an excellent source of fiber and may assist in the regulation of digestion.

6. COCONUT RICE PUDDING

INGREDIENTS:

- One cup of prepared white rice

- One cup of mild coconut milk

- Two tablespoons of honey

- One teaspoon of vanilla extract

STEPS:

1. Over medium heat, combine all ingredients in a saucepan.

2. Stir the mixture frequently until it thickens.

3. Serve either at room temperature or refrigerated.

Guidelines: For certain EPI patients, coconut milk is more digestible than dairy. Rice is a basic carbohydrate that is mild in the digestive system.

7. PEACH GELATIN

INGREDIENTS:

• One cup of peach juice (100% juice, no added sugar)

• One cup of water

• Two teaspoons of unflavored gelatin

• Sliced apricots for garnish

STEPS:

1. Heat water in a saucepan until it is tepid.

2. Add gelatin and stir until it is dissolved.

3. Incorporate peach juice.

4. Pour the mixture into molds and refrigerate until it has solidified.

5. Before serving, add sliced peaches as a garnish.

Gelatin is easily digestible, and peach juice offers vitamins and natural flavor. Guarantee that the beverage is devoid of any additional carbohydrates.

General Recommendations For Desserts That Are EPI-Friendly

1. Low to Moderate Fat: Opt for alternative milk and low-fat dairy products.

2. Natural Sweeteners: Instead of refined carbohydrates, employ honey, maple syrup, or fruit purees.

3. Ease of Digestibility: Select gelatin-based desserts, baked goods, and delicate fruits.

4. High Fiber: To facilitate digestion, include fruits and cereals.

5. Forget lactose: Opt for lactose-free or alternative milk products.

Individuals with EPI can relish delectable delicacies that correspond to their nutritional requirements by adhering to these recipes and guidelines.

CHAPTER NINE

7 Smoothie Procedural Recipes For Exocrine Pancreatic Insufficiency (EPI)

Careful dietary planning is necessary to manage symptoms and ensure adequate nutrition when living with Exocrine Pancreatic Insufficiency (EPI). Smoothies can be a convenient and nutritious alternative, providing a means of consuming essential nutrients that are gentle on the digestive system.

It is crucial to prioritize ingredients that are easily digestible, abundant in vitamins, and low in fat when creating smoothies for an EPI diet. The following are seven smoothie recipes that have been specifically designed to meet these criteria, along with the necessary guidelines to guarantee that they satisfy your dietary requirements.

EPI-Friendly Smoothies: A Guide

1. Minimal fat: Opt for ingredients that are either fat-free or minimal in fat. If dairy is employed, select low-fat or lactose-free alternatives.

2. High Protein: Incorporate protein-rich ingredients, such as Greek yogurt, cottage cheese, or protein supplements, to promote overall health and muscle maintenance.

3. Fiber: To facilitate digestion without causing discomfort, incorporate soluble fiber from fruits and vegetables.

4. Low Sugar: Use natural sweeteners such as maple syrup or honey sparingly and limit the addition of carbohydrates.

5. Digestive Enzymes: If your healthcare provider suggests it, you may want to add digestive enzyme supplements.

6. Hydration: Guarantee that you consume an adequate amount of fluids by consuming water or unsweetened beverages.

7. Balance: Strive to maintain energy levels by consuming a well-balanced combination of carbohydrates, proteins, and lipids.

Smoothie Recipes

1. BANANA BERRY BLAST

INGREDIENTS:

- One cup of frozen assorted fruit

- One mature banana

- One cup of low-fat Greek yogurt

- One cup of strained almond milk

- One tablespoon of honey (optional)

STEPS:

1. Combine all components in a blender.

2. Blend until the mixture is uniform.

3. If necessary, add more almond milk to achieve the desired consistency.

4. Serve immediately.

2. SMOOTHIE WITH GREEN POWER

INGREDIENTS:

- One cup of spinach leaves

- Sliced cucumber, 1/2 cup

- One green apple, cored and sliced

- One-half of an avocado

- One cup of coconut water

- The juice of half a lemon

STEPS:

1. Spinach, cucumber, apple, avocado, coconut water, and lemon juice should be combined in a blender.

2. Blend until the consistency is smooth.

3. Pour the beverage into a glass and savor it.

3. TROPICAL DELIGHT

INGREDIENTS:

- One cup of chilled mango segments

- 1/2 cup of pineapple segments

- One-half of a banana

- One cup of low-fat coconut milk

- One tablespoon of chia seeds

STEPS:

1. Combine mango, pineapple, banana, coconut milk, and chia seeds in a Vitamix.

2. Blend until the mixture is uniform.

3. Allow the chia seeds to expand by allowing them to settle for a few minutes.

4. Stir and serve.

4. SMOOTHIE MADE WITH OATMEAL

INGREDIENTS:

- 1/2 cup of rolled oats

- One cup of strained almond milk

- One mature banana

- One tablespoon of almond butter

- 1/2 teaspoon of cinnamon

- One teaspoon of vanilla extract

STEPS:

1. Soak cereals in almond milk for 5-10 minutes.

2. Incorporate the soaked oats, banana, almond butter, cinnamon, and vanilla into the blender.

3. Blend until the mixture is uniform.

4. Indulge in this breakfast for a satisfying meal.

5. SMOOTHIE WITH BERRIES AND SPINACH

INGREDIENTS:

- One cup of fresh spinach

- One cup of frozen assorted fruit

- One cup of low-fat Greek yogurt

- 1/2 cup of unsweetened almond milk or water

- One tablespoon of flaxseed grain

STEPS:

1. To the blender, add spinach, berries, yogurt, water or almond milk, and flaxseed meal.

2. Blend until the mixture is velvety and smooth.

3. Serve promptly for a refreshment that is rich in nutrients.

6. APPLE PIE SMOOTHIE

INGREDIENTS:

- One apple, cored and sliced

- 1/2 cup of low-fat cottage cheese

- One cup of strained almond milk

- One teaspoon of cinnamon

- One tablespoon of honey (optional)

- 1/2 teaspoon of vanilla extract

STEPS:

1. In a blender, combine almond milk, apple, cottage cheese, cinnamon, honey, and vanilla extract.

2. Blend until the mixture is uniform.

3. Indulge in a nutritious and comforting smoothie.

7. SMOOTHIE WITH CARROTS AND GINGER

INGREDIENTS:

- One cup of carrot juice

- 1/2 cup of pineapple segments

- One-half of a banana

- 1/2 teaspoon of freshly minced ginger

- One tablespoon of honey (optional)

STEPS:

1. Incorporate carrot juice, pineapple, banana, ginger, and honey into the blender.

2. Blend until the mixture is uniform.

3. Pour the beverage into a glass and savor the invigorating flavors.

In conclusion, smoothies are a beneficial and adaptable addition to an EPI diet, as they are mild on the digestive system and provide essential nutrients.

You can enjoy nutritious and delectable smoothies that promote your overall well-being and nutritional requirements by following the guidelines and experimenting with these recipes.

CHAPTER TEN

Maintaining A Healthy Lifestyle With EPI

Comprehending the condition and implementing the requisite lifestyle modifications are essential components of a fulfilling existence with EPI. This encompasses adhering to a particular diet, taking enzyme supplements as prescribed by your physician, and managing any symptoms that may arise. It is imperative to acquire knowledge regarding EPI and collaborate with your healthcare team to create a comprehensive management strategy that is customized to your requirements.

The Significance Of Consistent Medical Examinations

Individuals with EPI need to undergo routine medical examinations to monitor their condition and make any necessary modifications to their treatment plan.

Healthcare providers can promptly address any complications or changes in symptoms, evaluate digestive function, and assess enzyme levels during these check-ups. Individuals with EPI can more effectively manage their condition and maintain their overall health by maintaining regular appointments and remaining proactive.

Maintaining A Healthy Weight And Engaging In Physical Activity

Digestion and overall well-being can be substantially influenced by individuals with EPI who maintain a healthy weight and remain physically active. Digestion is stimulated by consistent exercise, which can mitigate symptoms such as bloating and discomfort.

Additionally, the risk of complications associated with EPI, including malnutrition and osteoporosis, is reduced by maintaining a healthy weight. Walking, swimming, or practicing yoga are straightforward exercises that can be advantageous and ought to be integrated into one's daily regimen.

Management Of Stress And Its Effect On Digestive Health

Symptoms of EPI can be exacerbated by stress, which can result in more discomfort and slower digestion. Stress management is imperative for individuals with EPI, and relaxation techniques such as meditation, yoga, or deep breathing are effective methods for management.

Reducing stress levels and enhancing overall digestion can be achieved by prioritizing self-care and identifying healthy coping mechanisms.

Additionally, the establishment of a supportive and tranquil atmosphere in both one's residence and workplace can enhance one's digestion and overall health.

Establishing A Support System

Individuals with EPI must establish a support system, as it offers practical assistance, encouragement, and emotional support when required. This support system may consist of online communities of individuals with similar experiences, healthcare providers, family, and acquaintances. The ability to communicate, share experiences, and rely on others during difficult periods can significantly impact the effective management of EPI. Support groups or counseling can also assist individuals in managing the emotional aspects of living with a chronic condition.

Monitoring And Modifying Your Diet Over Time

It is imperative to monitor and modify your diet over time to manage EPI and reduce symptoms. Working in conjunction with a registered dietitian or nutritionist is essential to develop a customized dietary plan that is tailored to your requirements and preferences. This may entail the avoidance of specific foods that exacerbate symptoms, such as high-fat or high-fiber choices, and the emphasis on easily digestible alternatives, such as lean proteins, prepared vegetables, and refined cereals.

Maintaining a food diary can assist in the identification of patterns and the tracking of triggers, thereby facilitating the more effective management of EPI symptoms.

Furthermore, it is crucial to periodically evaluate your diet and implement any required modifications to guarantee that you are achieving your nutritional requirements and preserving your health.

Conclusion

Exocrine Pancreatic Insufficiency (EPI) is a condition in which the pancreas fails to generate an adequate amount of digestive enzymes, resulting in nutrient deficiencies and malabsorption.

The management of EPI and the improvement of the quality of life for those affected are significantly influenced by their diet. The principal objective of an EPI diet is to guarantee sufficient nutrition while simultaneously alleviating symptoms such as abdominal pain, bloating, and diarrhea.

A well-organized EPI diet comprises small, frequent meals that are abundant in readily digestible nutrients. The emphasis is on the integration of complex carbohydrates, healthful lipids, and lean proteins.

To mitigate malnutrition and weight loss, patients frequently benefit from a high-calorie, nutrient-dense diet due to malabsorption issues. It is essential to supplement with pancreatic enzyme replacement therapy (PERT) with each meal to facilitate digestion and absorption.

In addition, the diet should be low in fiber to alleviate gastrointestinal distress and low in fat to alleviate the digestive burden, unless enzyme supplements are administered effectively. The inadequate assimilation of vitamins and minerals, particularly fat-soluble ones such as A, D, E, and K, in EPI patients may necessitate supplementation.

In summary, the management of EPI can be substantially improved by a tailored diet and appropriate enzyme supplementation, which can also reduce symptoms and improve nutritional status, thereby improving overall well-being. Consistent consultations with healthcare providers, including dietitians, are indispensable for the optimization of dietary strategies and the effective management of the condition.

THE END

www.ingramcontent.com/pod-product-compliance
Lightning Source LLC
Chambersburg PA
CBHW052325220526
45472CB00001B/275